THE
Little Book
of
Diet Help

THE
Little Book
of
Diet Help

Lose Weight—
Without Losing Your Mind

KIMBERLY WILLIS, PhD

ATRIA BOOKS

New York · *London* · *Toronto* · *Sydney* · *New Delhi*

ATRIA BOOKS

A Division of Simon & Schuster, Inc.
1230 Avenue of the Americas
New York, NY 10020

This publication contains the opinion and ideas of its author. It is intended to provide helpful and informational material on the subjects addressed in the publication. It is sold with the understanding that the author and publisher are not engaged in rendering medical, health, or any other kind of personal professional services in this book. The reader should consult his or her medical, health, or other competent professional before adopting any of the suggestions in this book or drawing inferences from it.

The author and publisher specifically disclaim all responsibility for any liability, loss, or risk, personal or otherwise, which is incurred as a consequence, directly or indirectly, of the use and application of any of the contents of this book.

First Atria Books hardcover edition December 2011

ATRIA BOOKS and colophon are trademarks of Simon & Schuster, Inc.

For information about special discounts for bulk purchases, please contact Simon & Schuster Special Sales at 1-866-506-1949 or business@simonandschuster.com.

The Simon & Schuster Speakers Bureau can bring authors to your live event. For more information or to book an event contact the Simon & Schuster Speakers Bureau at 1-866-248-3049 or visit our website at www.simonspeakers.com.

Illustrations copyright © Alexis Seabrook

Designed by Kyoko Watanabe

Manufactured in the United States of America

10 9 8 7 6 5 4 3 2 1

Library of Congress Control Number: 2011028299

ISBN 978-1-4516-6069-2
ISBN 978-1-4516-6070-8 (ebook)

For Mike
Who always believes in me

Contents

THE
Little Book
of
Diet Help

SECTION 1

About This Book

So you want to lose weight . . .

If you are reading this book you're probably no stranger to dieting.

The first thing you need to know is that this isn't a diet book. This book is different.

You already know what you need to do to lose weight.

Instead this book will help you shift the blocks that are stopping you from becoming your slimmer self.

This book will give you some knowledge about food and how it affects you—and as a result, you will find that you naturally begin to make changes in what you put into your body.

I will help you take control of your life, shed that unwanted weight, and become your best version of yourself.

The way this book differs from other weight-loss methods is that it will help you to adjust your attitudes to yourself, your body, and the food you eat by using exercises derived from yoga, acupressure, neuro-linguistic programming, and hypnotherapy.

These therapies are widely used around the world to help individuals deal with a variety of issues such as irrational anxieties, fears, stress, harmful habits, and a general lack of confidence.

You will find that by changing your thought patterns, your behavior will change—and when you reinforce those new, positive behaviors, you will start to free yourself of your negative habits and lose weight more easily and more permanently.

The exercises that I have decided to include in this book are ones that I have successfully used with my weight-loss groups. Individuals in those groups have found that through these exercises they changed their habits, felt more positive, more motivated, and ultimately lost weight more easily than when they had been on a restrictive diet.

Who am I?

I am a weight-loss specialist, and for many years I have worked with individuals and groups helping them become naturally slimmer, healthier, and happier with their bodies.

Most important, I am now here to help you. Today is the first day of the new you.

Kimberly Willis, PhD

What is keeping you attached to that excess weight?

Your past has emotional chains around you.

These chains stop you from moving forward.

They keep you attached to that excess weight.

Break these chains and you will find that you can let go of the weight you no longer need.

Working through the exercises in this book will help free you from the chains tying you to the past.

You will tap into your negative emotions by accessing powerful acupressure points. This will help break down the hold that these emotions have over you.

Your aim:

- To feel positive about yourself, your body, and how you look.
- To eat when you are hungry.
- To stop eating when you are no longer hungry.
- To free yourself from cravings.
- To feel motivated to exercise more.
- To lose weight easily and naturally.

Tapping explained

Within this book, you will find a number of "tapping" exercises, which are carried out on acupressure points throughout your body.

Some of these exercises are derived from EFT—Emotional Freedom Technique, developed by Gary Craig—which uses a specific set of acupressure points.

The theory behind this technique is that all emotional upsets are caused by disturbances in the body's energy system. Therefore, if you correct the energy disturbance, the emotional upset will disappear.

This is a very ancient practice, with deep historical roots. Around five thousand years ago, the Chinese discovered that pressing certain points on the body could help reduce pain. Using this knowledge, the Chinese went on to plot the energy lines of the body, known today as meridians. From this, the fields of acupressure and acupuncture were born.

Since then, the existence of energy lines within the body has been widely discussed and accepted as a tenet of many wellness therapies. Gently tapping along these meridians—while focusing on the issue that is bothering you—helps shift the energy in your body, settling the disturbances that are causing negative emotions to flare.

As a therapist I have seen firsthand how these techniques can result in amazing changes

After using one of the tapping exercises you may notice an instant change in how you feel. Or the effects may be more subtle: after a few days, you may look back over your recent behavior and realize that there has indeed been a positive shift in your actions.

Your tapping map

On the following pages, you'll find exercises that ask you to repeat specific affirmations, while tapping various pressure points on your body. To do this, follow the points on the diagram and tap each with your index and middle fingers about 8 times, saying the statement as you tap.

Begin by tapping your Karate Chop point, which is located on the side of your hand below your little finger, a soft fleshy area between your finger and wrist bone.

Move onto the inner eyebrow point, then the outer eyebrow point. Follow all the points on the face in the order they are numbered, while continuing to repeat the statement.

Now place your arm diagonally across your chest so that your fingers rest on your collarbone and tap this point.

Now you are ready to move onto the points on your hand. Using the opposite hand, tap on the side of each finger, next to the nail.

Continue to the Gamut point. This is located on the top of your hand, in the "V" that's created where the bones of your fourth and fifth fingers meet. Rub the skin in this "V" gently.

At the end of the sequence finish off by once again tapping the Karate Chop point.

Neuro-linguistic programming, NLP

This is a very complicated way of describing some of the easy techniques that are in this book. In essence, neuro-linguistic programming is about language, how we use it and how it affects us. It is also about our feelings and behavior.

NLP was developed by John Grinder and Richard Bandler in California in the 1970s. It harnesses the power of language to help you shift your views and beliefs.

You'll see it put into action in some of the easy techniques that are in this book.

For example, if you alter the tone of your voice as you repeat an affirmation, it can affect the way that you feel.

Or the way that you phrase something can affect your view of it:

> *"I am trying to lose weight, but it's hard."*

Becomes: *"Each and every day it's becoming easier to lose weight."*

In both of these cases neuro-linguistic programming is at work.

NLP can help you shift to a new viewpoint.

SECTION 2

Getting Started

QUICK METABOLISM BOOSTER

Deep belly breathing boosts your metabolism—and when your metabolism is boosted, you are burning more calories.

- Stand up.

- Place one hand on your stomach.

- Breathe deeply and slowly, through your nose, as if you could breathe into the depths of your stomach.

- Repeat for 5 breaths.

Remember:

Zero fat

does not mean

zero calories

Calories matter!

Feeling hungry?

Before reaching for a snack, have a glass of water.

When you are thirsty your body can send out hunger signals, because it knows that you can get water from food.

Drink some water and you might find that your hunger disappears.

Q: How can you burn more calories watching TV at night?

A: Exercise in the morning!

This will boost your metabolism for the rest of the day.

Even when you are sitting in front of the TV in the evening you will be burning more calories than normal.

UNWANTED FOOD CRAVING?

Rub the area between your nose and your top lip with your index finger for about a minute.

This is a soothing point that will comfort you and reduce your craving.

Hug someone!

When you hug someone you feel better.

When you feel better you eat better.

So go on—have a cuddle.

THE TEMPTATION BATTLE

Sometimes it feels like a battle is going on in your mind. A part of you knows you are not hungry and really don't want that cookie—but the other part of you is trying to convince yourself that it's okay to eat it—that after all, you deserve it.

Win the temptation battle!

If you find yourself tempted by snack food—like a bag of chips, a handful of M&Ms, or a late-night bowl of ice cream—try this exercise:

Touch the front part of your ear, that bit of cartilage that sticks out in front of your ear canal. Now, rub it between your thumb and index finger for a few minutes.

This is a strong acupressure point. Rubbing it will help turn off cravings by redirecting your energy and lowering your appetite.

The chemicals at work in your body: insulin

Insulin is a hormone produced by your body, which allows it to absorb sugar. Here's how it works:

- Insulin is produced by the pancreas to absorb sugar from your bloodstream.

- Refined carbohydrates, which are essentially sugars, are quickly absorbed into your bloodstream after a meal.

- After you eat a large amount of refined carbohydrates, your body rushes to produce enough insulin to absorb the high level of sugars in your blood.

- But when your blood-sugar levels inevitably drop you will probably feel hungry, irritable, and cranky.

The white carbohydrates and sugar hunger trap

Imagine a small child who has just eaten a huge bag of candy. You know what happens next—his energy will skyrocket and you'll practically have to peel him off the ceiling! Then before you know it, he'll crash—and he'll be irritable, unhappy, and likely to throw a tantrum. The same thing happens to adults when we eat processed foods—only instead of having a tantrum, we tend to reach for more comfort foods. Here's how the chemistry works:

When you eat a bowl of pasta or a slice of cake. . . .

- Your blood sugar zooms up.
- Your body releases more and more insulin to cope with the sudden increase.
- This excess insulin now causes your blood-sugar levels to plummet.
- As a result you feel hungry, tired, and irritable.
- You crave more food.
- You gain weight.
- More important, this can lead to type 2 diabetes.*

*As discussed in "Increased consumption of refined carbohydrates and the epidemic of type 2 diabetes in the United States: an ecologic assessment," by Lee S. Gross, Li Li, Earl S. Ford, and Simin Liu, *American Journal of Clinical Nutrition,* Vol. 79, No. 5, 774–779, May 2004.

How can you stabilize your blood sugar?

Eating protein (eggs, turkey, chicken) or unrefined carbohydrates (that's brown pasta, brown rice, and whole wheat or multigrain bread) prevents your blood-sugar levels from plummeting, instead causing a more gradual rise in blood-sugar levels.

When you stabilize your blood sugar:

- You feel fuller for longer.
- You eat less.
- You have more energy.
- You feel happier.
- You naturally lose weight.

Slim people stop eating when they are no longer hungry.

Overweight people stop eating when they are full.

AFTERNOON ENERGY BOOST

It's 4 p.m. You are tired, and you need an energy boost.

Try this exercise as an alternative to going to the vending machine.*

- Stand up.

- Start marching, lifting your knees high and swinging the opposite arms.

- Now shift to marching with the same-side arms and legs moving together.

- Repeat for a minute or two.

*An applied kinesiology technique.

Beware, beware the bliss point . . .

This is a special point in your brain that is stimulated by foods containing excessive amounts of **fat, salt, and sugar**.

Think pizzas, cookies, and battered chicken.

Your brain loves it when this point is stimulated—it's like a drug, and your brain doesn't want this feeling to end.

Part of your brain is going to try to keep you eating more and more of this food.

Even if you are full—stuffed—it will still want you to eat more.

When the bliss point takes over, you just can't stop eating. You are out of control.*

Be aware of the foods that trigger this for you—this is what some manufacturers work toward. They want you to crave more and more of their product. **Avoid those foods—they will beat any willpower!**

If you recognize this behavior, then you need to avoid the foods that cause it.

---

*As discussed in the excellent book *The End of Overeating* by David A. Kessler.

Is all hunger the same?

Physical Hunger   Comes hours after your last meal. This is a real hunger— one that you need to pay attention to.

Emotional Hunger   Is caused by a negative or positive emotional trigger and can hit you any time of the day, even if you have just eaten. *This type of hunger makes you gain weight.*

POSITIVE MIND AND
BODY BOOST

This exercise will help you to feel good and to reconnect with your body.

- Stand up.

- Bring your hands in front of your chest in prayer position. As you inhale deeply, raise your hands, still in prayer position, above your head and look up.

- Hold this position as you inhale and exhale deeply for a couple of breaths. On your next out breath, bring your hands back in front of your chest. Repeat 3 times.

- Each time you raise your hands, feel yourself rooting into the ground as you simultaneously stretch toward the sky.

- Finish by tapping the top of your head with your fingertips, like raindrops. Notice how much calmer and lighter you feel.

As you go about your day, periodically tune into your body, and recall the sensation of peace and ease that you felt as you finished this exercise.

Remember:
When you feel better you eat better.

Eat better

Forget about eating right

Eating better is easier than eating right.*

Eating right all the time can be hard work and depressing. Plus, you will probably fail—and when you do, you will then feel that much worse.

You can succeed at eating better than you have before. You can feel good about yourself and the positive changes that you are making.

When you fail at eating right, you will feel bad. When you feel bad you are more likely to comfort eat. This is what restrictive diets do to you.

Eating better makes you feel good. It's about the many small accomplishments that add up to a big change. Most important, it allows you to be human—and humans make mistakes!

*As discussed in *Mindless Eating* by Brian Wansink, New York: Bantam, 2010.

Eat slowly!

Chew slowly!

Pay attention to what you are eating.

Binge eaters don't taste
what they are eating.

Notice your food. Smell your food.

Chew slowly. Savor the tastes and
textures of each mouthful.

Appreciate your food.

Stop forbidding certain foods

Why should you? Try this:

Don't think of pink elephants.

I'll bet you did!

Now say to yourself, "I'm not having chocolate, no chocolate, no chocolate."

What does your brain hear?

Chocolate Chocolate **Chocolate Chocolate**

This will beat even the strongest willpower. Because you were so fixated on forbidding chocolate, it was all you could think about—and you ate a pound of it.

Instead, allow yourself a bit of chocolate and open up your thoughts and your energy for other, better things.

Are you hungry?

Put your hand on your stomach and notice how your stomach is really feeling.

Ignoring real physical hunger until you are starving causes your body to slow down, as it thinks there is a famine and it must save energy.

When this happens, you stop burning calories.

Then when you do eat, your body is worried that this might be all the food there is, and it will store reserves (on your stomach and butt) and make you eat extra, just in case there is another famine on the way.

So when you are hungry—EAT!

And place your hand on your stomach once
an hour, just to see how it is feeling.

You have probably been ignoring your stomach
for years—it could do with a bit of attention.

Eat slowly.

Eat with awareness.

Stop eating when you are
no longer hungry.

Feel that excess weight melt away.

. . . It really is that simple.

Are all calories the same?

NO!

Rate at which food leaves your stomach:

- Protein: around 4 calories per minute
- Sugar and carbohydrates: up to 30 calories per minute

This means:

Eating high-protein foods will keep you fuller for longer, as they take more time for your stomach to digest.

As a result, you will eat less and lose more weight.

The chemicals at work in your body: serotonin

Serotonin is a neurotransmitter, which is made in your body from tryptophan.

Serotonin is responsible for your "happy feeling." It also helps regulate moods, causing you to feel calmer and to sleep well.

Low serotonin levels have been linked to feeling *emotionally* low.

Eating refined carbohydrates will result in a short-term boost in serotonin, but the pleasure this leads to will quickly disappear as your blood-sugar levels rapidly drop, leaving you feeling tired and down.

To maintain stable levels of serotonin it is important to eat foods containing tryptophan—salmon, turkey, almonds, bananas, avocados, eggs, and also complex carbohydrates, like oatmeal or whole wheat.

If dieting in the past has left you feeling melancholy or unhappy, it's probably because you weren't taking proper care of your serotonin levels. When you begin to change your diet, it is important that you support your body with things that will promote both your physical and mental well-being.

Real mood boosters

Serotonin is a chemical in the brain that triggers positive emotions. But it also exists in large quantities in the gut. There is a complex relationship between the stomach and the brain, which makes it very important to look after your body's serotonin levels.

You can start by paying attention to the foods you are eating, as some contain tryptophan. Your body needs tryptophan in order to make serotonin, so there are literally some foods that can boost your mood and your energy.

There are other ways, besides food, to boost your serotonin levels.

Exercise
Sleep
Spending time with friends
Pets
Sunlight
Positive thoughts

All these make you feel better, and as a result you will eat better—and be more motivated to look after your body.

Take care
with
aspartame

Aspartame can deplete your serotonin levels, causing you to feel down. *

As a result, you might crave comfort foods and fall into the trap of emotional eating.

Since many low-fat and low-calorie foods contain aspartame, beware—this is one of the ways that some so-called "diet foods" can lead to weight gain.

*As discussed in "Direct and indirect cellular effects of aspartame on the brain," by P. Humphries, E. Pretorius, and H. Naude, *European Journal of Clinical Nutrition,* Vol. 62, No. 4, 451–462, May 2008.

Remember:

Protein stabilizes blood sugar
and reduces your appetite;
it will reduce the amount
of food you eat in a day.

Good sources of protein include
grilled chicken, eggs, fish, tofu,
almonds, pumpkin seeds, beans.

Listen Listen Listen

Listen to your body: when it is
physically hungry—eat.

When you eat, choose something
good for your body.

Your body will believe that
there is plenty of food, and your
metabolism will speed up.

Changing How You Feel

How you feel

. . . affects your body.
. . . affects your metabolism and your energy levels.
. . . affects what you eat.
. . . affects how effectively you will exercise.

When you are trying to lose weight, stress
is the enemy working against you.

Learning how you can make yourself feel calmer
and happier is essential for long-term weight loss.

Would you say that to a friend?

Notice what you say to yourself during the day.

You are probably saying horrible things.

Start to break the habit of being mean to yourself.

Break the habit of making yourself feel bad.

Negative thoughts drain your emotional and physical energy.

If you feel sad, anxious, alone, or incapable, you are more likely to turn to comfort food.

Think about something that you like about yourself.

Interrupt those bad thoughts.

Stress

The only explanation that your body has for stress is FAMINE.

So when you are stressed, your body will slow your metabolism down to save on food, thinking . . .

"Famine is coming—better stock up!"

Finding ways to reduce your stress levels will help keep your metabolism working at its optimum level—which will ultimately help you lose weight.

Try introducing a few minutes of a calming exercise like mindfulness into your day.

What is mindfulness?

Mindfulness is a way of being present in the moment.

Being present in the moment means not trying to change anything; it means simply being aware.

Many of us are so busy—always thinking about what happened yesterday, and what we need to accomplish tomorrow—that we forget about the moment that we're in. We forget about *now*.

Being aware of *now* is about being present in a non-judgmental way.

It's a simple practice that can have big effects.

Brain time

Practice mindfulness

When you practice mindfulness—even for just a few minutes a day—you are allowing your head some recovery time. You are giving your busy brain the chance to adjust and rebalance.

Mindfulness will help you become free of the comfort foods you rely on to numb and soothe anxious thoughts.

Quieting your mind also allows it to reconnect with your body.

MINDFULNESS

Just 5 minutes of mindfulness a day will calm your mind and body, reduce stress, and make you feel happier. When your mind and body are more at peace, you will feel better and eat better.

- Sit or lie down. Close your eyes.

- Starting from the top of your head, mentally scan through your body, taking the time to notice how you are physically feeling. What parts are comfortable or uncomfortable?

- Now, in a nonjudgmental way, notice how you are feeling emotionally. Are you grumpy, calm, stressed, happy, sad?

- Start to focus your breathing. Inhale and exhale deeply, in and out of your nose, as if you could breathe into the depths of your stomach.

- After focusing on your breathing for a minute or two, take a deep breath in, and as you exhale, imagine the number one in your mind. You may see it in your mind's eye, or imagine that you can hear it.

- With your next out breath imagine the number two. Continue counting with each exhale up to ten, and then start again with one.

- As you count, keep your eyes closed and remain comfortably seated or lying down.

- Continue counting from one to ten for 5 or 10 minutes.

As you do this you may find your mind drifting away. If you realize this is happening, just gently pull your mind back to counting and focusing on your breath. This will become easier with practice.

Beliefs are very powerful

What do you believe?

- I have always failed at diets.
- I am always going to be big.
- I have a slow metabolism.
- It is hard to lose weight at my age.
- I have no willpower.
- I just can't lose weight.

What is your strongest negative belief about your body and your weight?

Think about the power that this belief has over you.

Your mind works very hard to make your beliefs come true.

TAPPING OUT NEGATIVE BELIEFS

Helping you break free of the thoughts
that are weighing you down

Focus on one specific negative belief. Follow the
points on the tapping map and do one full circuit for
each affirmation. Repeat each statement out loud as
you tap.

For further reference, please see the tapping map on page 9.

- Even though I have this belief, I am okay.

- Even though I believe that this is true, I am okay.

- I know that this belief began for a reason, but it is in the past now, and I can move on.

- I can allow myself to imagine what it would be like to let this belief go.

- I can allow myself to imagine what it would feel like if this belief weren't true.

- This makes me feel _____ (energized, free, powerful, unburdened).

MOOD BOOSTER

Remember: when you feel better, you eat better, and you exercise more.

This is an easy mood booster to use when you feel a bit low.

- Stand up.

- Breathe deeply.

- Look up toward the sky.

- Stretch your hands up above your head, spreading your fingers apart.

- Smile (even if you don't feel like it).

- Smile (go on, show those teeth!).

- Smile at the world.

- As you exhale gently, lower your hands and shake them out.

Being able to change your
mood is very important.

Recognize that you are in
charge of your mood.

Your mood can determine
your metabolism.

Your mood affects what you eat.

How does your mood affect your metabolism?

When you are in a good mood your serotonin levels are likely to be high.

Not only do higher levels of serotonin benefit your overall happiness, they also suppress your appetite, causing you to eat small regular meals.

This type of eating boosts your metabolism.

When you are in a bad mood, it is likely that your serotonin levels are lower.

This will probably cause you to crave refined carbohydrates, as they provide a short-term serotonin boost.

You will probably eat a large meal—and then nothing for several hours.

Your metabolism will slow down, as there is no food to process. As a result, you will also start to feel tired.

You will exercise less, which will in turn contribute to your metabolic slowdown.

GROUNDING AND BREATHING

This quick exercise will help when you are feeling anxious or stressed. When your thoughts seem to be spinning around, you can use this technique to provide on-the-spot calming.

* Stand up and notice the weight of your feet on the ground. Make sure your knees are loose—not locked.

* Imagine that your feet are really planted into the ground, like the roots of a tall strong oak tree.

* Now, allow your shoulders to relax gently, away from your ears.

* Place one hand on your belly, and breathe deeply into the depths of your stomach. Imagine that this point, a couple of inches below your navel, is the very core of you.

* This is your navel center or chakra, a center of emotional well-being and the spot where much of the body's good energy or ch'i is stored.

* Stay in this position for a few breaths.

This exercise is good for instant soothing of mind and body.

Your unconscious mind is always working to make you happy

But sometimes, it gets it wrong.

For example, your unconscious mind wants you to feel happy and it knows that chocolate can do this. So it makes you crave chocolate when you are feeling down. What it doesn't know is that this is just a short-term fix. Relying on chocolate when you're feeling sad or anxious will, in reality, make you gain weight—and ultimately, this will only make you unhappier.

Your mind needs to be reeducated—it needs to learn new ways of making you feel better.

Becoming more aware of how your deeper mind is working against you means that you are already starting to make changes.

Stop pretending that your body isn't there

It is—and it's time you took some notice of it.

Are you drawing an invisible line at your neck—and ignoring what's below it?

You are not wearing an Elizabethan collar! Look down—your body is waiting.

Pay attention to it!

If you want to make changes to how your body looks you are going to have to start acknowledging that it is there.

How are you? (Yes, YOU)

Tune into your body.
Reconnect with your body.

Do something nice for it,

take a bubble bath,

lather on some lovely skin cream,

get a pedicure,

care for yourself.

When you care for your body you are more likely to take care of what you put *into* your body.

Love your body

"The curious paradox is that when I accept myself just as I am, then I can change."

—CARL ROGERS, AMERICAN PSYCHOLOGIST

If you hate your body and tell it so constantly, then it won't want to work with you to lose weight. Not to mention that you will be exhausted from this constant battle with yourself.

Showing love and acceptance to your body has energizing effects. It enables it to work with you to create a slimmer, happier you.

LOVING YOUR BODY

This uses a yoga position that links the heart and navel chakras. The navel chakra boosts feelings of confidence and self-esteem, while the heart chakra inspires love and kindness. Encouraging these wonderful, positive feelings within you will help you to love and care for your beautiful body.

- Close your eyes.

- With your fingertips, gently tap the points on the inside edge of your eyebrows, then the outside edge of your eyebrows, and finally, tap below your eyes. Tap about eight times on each point.

- As you do this, take deep breaths and think about your body—the amazing things it has allowed you to do, the places it has taken you, the people you have met.

- Keeping your eyes closed, place your right hand on your heart and your left hand on your stomach, below your belly button. Think appreciative, kind, and loving thoughts toward your body.

- As you breathe deeply, imagine the air from your inhaled breath flowing from your heart down into your belly, and back again as you exhale.

MORNING ENERGY BOOST

Get in the habit of doing this exercise in the shower every morning. It will give you a quick and easy energy boost, and start you on the right path for your day ahead.

Using both of your hands, lightly tap each of these points for about 30 seconds with your fingertips:

- Just below the points on your collarbone. (1, 2)

- Along the center of your sternum. (3)

- At the bottom of your ribs, in line with the nipples. (4, 5)

- Finally tap all over the top of your head, like raindrops.

- Shake out your hands.

These are strong acupressure points that will boost your well-being.*

*An adaptation of Donna Eden's Triple Thump, in her *Energy Medicine for Women* (New York: Tarcher, 2008).

How do you want to look?

What does reaching your goal look like?

Toned | **Slim** | **Healthy** | **Gorgeous** | **Fit** | **Strong**

Now, be honest: when you see others who are already at this weight, how do you describe them?

Small | **Scrawny** | **Ditzy** | **Haggard** | **Pathetic**

> Your mind will not let you achieve
> something you feel is negative.

If you are thinking negative thoughts toward slimmer people, start changing the message.

Turn it into something that your mind will want to achieve.

Who is the fairest of them all?

What happens when you look in the mirror?

Do you focus on the parts of your body that you hate?

What horrible thoughts are you thinking toward your body?

You need to get your body on your side. Look in the mirror and apologize to your body.

Yes, this is going to feel silly— but you really need to get your body working for you!

Now say something nice to your body. Look in the mirror and focus on a part of your body that you like. Perhaps it's your lovely hair, your beautiful eyes, or your slim ankles. Recognize the good that already exists in your figure.

You are the fairest of them all.

When you are being kinder to your body you will automatically take more care with what you put into it.

How do I look?

Close your eyes and imagine that you are standing naked in front of a full-length mirror.

When you hear that inner voice making those negative comments:

- **Repeat the comments out loud in a silly voice like Donald Duck.**
- **Answer the comments back—be strong, be confident.**
- **Now start to repeat the opposite comment to yourself—make that negative a positive!**

Example: "You have fat legs—you look awful in slacks."

Now becomes: "I look great in slacks—my legs are becoming slimmer every day."

Begin to take more notice of that negative inner voice—it is chipping away at your self-esteem. As you recognize it you will take away its power over you.

Stop avoiding your
own reflection.

Make the mirror your
friend—not your enemy.

TAPPING AWAY THE POWER OF THE MIRROR

Helping you feel more confident
in your appearance

Follow the points on the tapping map and do one full
circuit for each affirmation. Repeat each statement
out loud as you tap.

For further reference, please see the tapping map on page 9.

- I accept myself and how I look.

- I can allow myself to say nice things about how I look.

- I can look in the mirror and focus on the things I like about myself.

- I can allow myself to accept compliments.

- I can choose to stop making myself feel bad.

- I have the power to make myself feel good.

WHO APPRECIATES YOU?

This exercise will help you to feel compassionate toward yourself.

Think about someone in your life who appreciates you just as you are.

Close your eyes for a few moments and imagine that person is standing in front of you, smiling and telling you that you are wonderful.

Let yourself accept those positive thoughts—soak up the warmth of them, and keep that positive glow with you all day.

Feel that love and appreciation for who you are.

The brain in your stomach

You have neurons in your stomach—this is why you can literally feel emotions in your gut.

So negative feelings—like anxiety, dread, sadness—register in the pit of your stomach.

Eating is a way that we try to push down and cover up these negative emotions.

Even though it can be scary sometimes, it is okay to face these negative thoughts and work through them.

When you deal with them you can begin to let them go.

You can be free of these negative emotions, which are causing you to eat much more than you need.

It might be that you need some positive emotional input.

The first step to being kind to your heart and mind is to look after your body.

Become aware of just how important you are.

In order to gain control you must take responsibility for yourself

- It is not your mother's fault you are overweight.
- It is not your partner's fault you are overweight.
- It is not your job's fault you are overweight.
- It is not your kid's fault you are overweight.
- It is not the dog's fault that you are overweight.

It is your fault.

This means you have the power to do something about it.

Because if it's not your fault, you are powerless, and that isn't something you want to be. When you take responsibility for yourself, your body, and your emotions, you have the ability to change them.

You have power and
control over your life.

In order to have control
of your life, your body,
your weight,

you must take responsibility
for yourself.

Only then can you
make changes.

When you are
responsible, you
are in control.

Control

Are you willing to give control of your life over to others?

Taken to the extreme, this can lead to depression and illness.

When you reclaim control, you are letting go of blame that you have put on others for all the things that have happened to you.

When you take control you have the power to change.

This can feel scary—but it can also feel energizing, fantastic, and wonderful.

BREATHING FOR CALM

This yoga exercise quickly calms your mind and can help restore balance to your busy life. It will relax you and reduce stress, enabling you to avoid comfort eating, and instead eat for health.

- Stand or sit comfortably.

- Inhale through your nostrils and exhale slowly through your mouth.

- Exaggerate your breathing as you exhale, making a "haaaaaa" sound. Feel this sound reverberate at the back of your throat.

- Repeat several times.

- As you are exhaling, notice yourself letting go of heavy stresses and worries, letting your shoulders drop a little each time.

- As you inhale, imagine breathing in a light, calm feeling.

Stress changes your brain chemistry

When all else in life is chaos, the one thing you have control over is what you are going to put into your body.

This is another reason why you can find yourself turning to food for comfort.

It is this control aspect of food that can also lead to eating disorders.

Remember that you are the boss of what you eat.

You need to teach your mind and body that there are better ways to lower stress.

The chemicals at work in your body: cortisol

When your body is under stress it releases extra amounts of a hormone called cortisol.

This is the same hormone that triggers your body's "fight or flight" response.

Evolutionarily speaking, this is very important. But when your body experiences long-term exposure to high levels of cortisol, there are negative effects:

- Higher blood pressure
- Decrease in muscle tissue
- Lowered immunity
- Decrease in bone density
- Altered blood-sugar levels
- Decreased fertility
- Reduced serotonin levels

Your brain under stress

If you want to lose weight and keep it off, you'll need to learn how to reduce your stress levels.

- Stress increases the levels of cortisol in the brain.
- This can cause you to crave comfort foods.
- Comfort foods will seem to dull the stress for a short time.
- But these same comfort foods also lead to an overproduction of insulin—and as a result, your blood-sugar levels will soon begin to plunge.
- You will feel tired and irritable and crave more comfort food.
- You will gain weight.

Remember: Practicing mindfulness can help to dramatically reduce your stress levels.

SECTION 4

Understanding
Your Food Rules

Your food rules

You live your life by a series of rules or habits. You brush your teeth in the morning. You call your mother on Thursdays. Once a month you have a girls' night out.

You also have food rules—patterns and habits that your mind has programmed in and that you now perform automatically.

What are your food rules?

- I always have cereal and toast in the morning.
- I always have pizza on a Friday night.
- I always have a muffin with a cup of coffee.
- I always get popcorn when I see a film.
- I always eat everything on my plate.

Are your food rules ruling you?

Learning about your own food rules is a crucial component of changing the way you look, as these are the habits that may be keeping you stuck where you are.

Breaking your rules

Make a list of your current food rules.

Now make a separate list of some new alternatives that you would be happier with.

I always have a muffin with a cup of coffee

becomes

I choose to have a piece of fruit with my coffee.

Be aware of your old rules, and begin to implement the new ones.

The first time you make a change it may feel difficult, but each time after this it will become easier and easier.

TAPPING INTO YOUR ABILITY
TO CREATE BETTER FOOD RULES

Helping you break free of your negative patterns

Follow the points on the tapping map and do one full circuit for each affirmation. Repeat each statement out loud as you tap.

For further reference, please see the tapping map on page 9.

- Even though I don't think I can change my food rules, I am okay.

- Even though it feels hard to change, I accept myself.

- (Rubbing the "sore spot," described on page 120), I have always done this, and it feels as if I always will.

- (Returning to the tapping map) Even though I can't imagine doing something different, I am okay.

- Even if this won't help me to change my food rules, I accept myself.

- Even though it's hard to let go of this excess weight that's stopping me from having the life I want, I accept myself.

Beware the clean plate club

No lives were ever saved by those who

cleared all the food off their plate.

When you are no longer hungry . . .

STOP EATING

A MOMENT OF CALM

Sometimes there just aren't enough hours in the day for quality "me time." This two-minute exercise will give your mind and body a quick boost, calming you and allowing you to put life into perspective.

- Place your right hand on your heart.

- Place your left hand on your stomach, just below your belly button.

- Close your eyes and breathe deeply through your nose.

- Gently drop your shoulders away from your ears.

- Send yourself a compliment:

    "I am a good friend." "I am a caring mother."
    "I work hard." "I am an honest person."

- Bask in this compliment for a few moments before opening your eyes and going on with your day.

FOOD CRAVING BREAK

Do you find yourself craving a specific food?

Try doing this exercise to break down the strength of that craving:

- Place your right hand on the center of your chest.

- Rub the skin between the bones of the fourth and fifth fingers of your right hand, the Gamut point, with the fingers of your left hand.

- As you rub this point, focus your mind on the food that you have been craving.

Stimulating these acupressure points helps to calm the mind and reduce the craving.

Are you having constant cravings?

Have you been ignoring physical hunger? Skipping meals?

If so, your body will start craving foods that will give it a fast sugar boost.

Remember, if you eat refined sugars and carbohydrates your blood sugar will only temporarily lift before crashing—leaving you feeling tired, low, irritable, and craving more food.

As a result you will eat more than you need—and inevitably, you will gain weight.

You have a choice.

> **Change your routine.**

>> **Interrupt the cycle.**

>>> **Have a new plan.**

TAPPING ON CRAVINGS—BREAK DOWN THOSE ATTACHMENTS

Helping you separate emotion from food

Follow the points on the tapping map and do one full circuit for each affirmation. Repeat each statement out loud as you tap.

For further reference, please see the tapping map on page 9.

- Even though I have a craving, I am okay.

- Even though I really want to eat _____, I am okay.

- Even though I don't want to give up this food, I accept myself.

- Even though I don't feel I can give up this craving, I am okay.

- This food helps me in some way.

- It makes me feel better.

- Even though I do not feel I have control over this craving, I am okay.

- Even though I can't imagine what I will do without this food, I accept myself, and that feels good.

Finish by using both hands to tap across the top of your head, as if your fingertips were raindrops.

QUICK CRAVING TAP

When you find yourself standing in the kitchen deciding whether or not you are going to give in to a craving, this exercise will help you make a quick emotional shift.*

Begin tapping at your temple, following the skin behind the ears and down the sides of your neck, ending as you reach the tops of your shoulders.

Left-hand side:

As you tap, repeat this phrase 5 times:

I no longer like the taste of _____.

Right-hand side:

As you tap, repeat this phrase 5 times:

I love being free from craving _____.

*Developed by George Goodheart, the founder of applied kinesiology, and Donna Eden, author of Energy Medicine for Women.

When do you overeat?

Make a list of the times, situations, or places at which you regularly overeat.

Now come up with a new plan—write down something else that you could do in each scenario, something that would make you feel better about yourself.

It's easier to make a plan when you are not in the moment.

Now, when that situation next arises you can choose to do something else that will make you feel good. Your mind will already have an alternative route that it can choose to follow.

CRAVING COMFORT FOOD?

Try this if you are feeling low and craving comfort food.

- Rub the area of skin just below the nail on the little finger of your left hand.

- Gently rub from the side of the nail, near the ring finger, to the outside edge of the nail

- Repeat this action for a minute.

This is a strong acupressure point and can help to ease low moods.

TAPPING OUT YOUR ATTACHMENT TO COMFORT FOODS

Helping you break out of a cycle of emotional eating

Follow the points on the tapping map and do one full circuit for each affirmation. Repeat each statement out loud as you tap.

For further reference, please see the tapping map on page 9.

- Even though I comfort eat, I accept myself.

- Even though I have done this for so long, I am okay.

- Even though I am worried that I won't be able to stop comfort eating, I am okay.

- It's scary to imagine life without comfort eating.

- I can't imagine choosing to do something else.

- It could feel good to let this comfort eating go.

- I can allow myself to be free of comfort eating—it was an old habit that I no longer need.

"There aren't enough cookies
in the world to make you
feel loved and whole."

—MICHAEL NEILL,
BESTSELLING AUTHOR AND LIFE COACH
WWW.SUPERCOACH.COM

Overcoming Emotional Eating

TURNING OFF EMOTIONAL HUNGER

This exercise will activate the energy in your stomach and allow your mind to be aware of how it is feeling, helping you to distinguish between physical and emotional hunger.

- Stand comfortably with your arms by your sides.

- Slowly lift your arms. When they are above your head, reach back as far as is comfortable. Feel the stretch in your stomach before returning to a neutral, upright position.

- Slowly lower your arms. Repeat three times.

Take care with this exercise if you have back problems.

Food Cravings = Emotional Hunger

TAPPING OUT EMOTIONAL EATING

Begin tapping at your temple, following the skin behind the ears and down the sides of your neck, and ending as you reach the tops of your shoulders.*

Left-hand side:

As you tap, repeat this phrase 5 times:

Negative feelings no longer cause me to overeat.

Right-hand side:

As you tap, repeat this phrase 5 times:

I eat for a slim and healthy body.

*Developed by George Goodheart, the founder of applied kinesiology, and Donna Eden, author of *Energy Medicine for Women*.

Extend your view

Imagine you are looking at some very tempting, highly fattening food.

> You want it, you deserve it, you need a
> bit—after all, it's been a hard week.

It's really easy to talk yourself into eating it.

But you are only thinking about the next 30 seconds of your life.

Now—imagine your perspective is changing.

Think about how you'll feel 30 minutes from now. Now envision yourself in 30 days.

> What do you want to be doing?
> What do you want to be wearing?

Think about how this type of food will stop you from achieving your goal.

Now the food becomes less appealing, even disgusting. You see it for what it really is: momentary pleasure but long-term sabotage, which will only lead to guilt and a sense of failure.

> How different does that food look
> when you see the real outcome?

> You can choose not to eat it, and feel
> satisfied as a result. You can choose.

The diet tightrope

As you learn new techniques to help you lose weight and to make changes in your life that will keep the weight off for good, you are also letting go of that stressful diet tightrope you used to try and balance on.

You are now walking along a new path, and it's one that allows you to make some mistakes.

When you slip up—and you will, because you are only human—it no longer means falling off that tightrope. Instead, you are just wandering from side to side on a new, wider path before you straighten out again.

What does this mean?

It means that when you have some chocolate now, you have a little bit. You don't feel that huge sense of failure and then simply succumb to it by eating the entire bar. Now, you can enjoy a small piece and put the rest away.

Some days you will fail.

Expect it. Accept it. You are
only human. It is okay.

Forgive yourself.

CRAVING BLASTER

Use this exercise when you just can't seem to break free from a craving—and it's driving you nuts!*

* Stand up.

* Put your arms out in front of you, palms up; bend your elbows and make your hands into fists.

* Think about the craving you want to let go of.

* As you inhale deeply, swing your arms up behind and above your head.

* As you loudly exhale, swing your arms back down in front of you—opening up your hands, with your palms facing upward.

* Repeat three times.

* End by placing one hand on your heart and the other on your belly. Close your eyes and take three deep breaths, inhaling and exhaling through your nose.

* You will find yourself feeling happier, lighter, and freer.

*Derived from Donna Eden's Blow-out technique, *Energy Medicine for Women* (New York: Tarcher, 2008).

SECTION 6

Looking after Your Liver

Your personal washing machine

Your liver is your body's washing machine.

The liver's job is to cleanse toxins from the body.

But the liver has to prioritize the toxins it deals with.

If there is alcohol in the body, the liver targets that first.

When your liver is busy absorbing alcohol, it cannot process the excess fat that you have been trying so hard to get rid of.

As a result, you don't lose any weight.

Alcohol wears
your body out

(And keeps you out of the clothes you want to wear.)

Alcohol raises the levels of cortisol—the stress hormone—in your body.

Excessive levels of cortisol can lead to sleep problems and a decrease in muscle mass.

In turn, poor sleep causes further hormone imbalances, which can increase your appetite and desire for comfort foods.

Alcohol can cause you to lose muscle mass and to eat more food.

It's just a drink . . .

When alcohol comes into the body, the liver breaks it down.

Alcohol intake reduces the liver's ability to remove fat from your blood, and also causes it to increase its production of triglycerides.

An excess of triglycerides can be stored as fat in the liver. This could result in fatty liver disease.

Fatty deposits in your liver also reduce its efficiency in removing toxins from your body.

Excessive amounts of triglycerides in the body can also increase the risk of strokes and heart attacks.

When your body is busy processing alcohol, it's not processing food or fat.

The result? You don't lose any weight.

A fatty belly can mean a fatty liver

Excess body fat is often indicative of an overworked liver.

Things that tire out a liver:

Alcohol | **Sugar** | **Caffeine** | **Processed foods**

Refined carbohydrates | **Fatty foods**

Go on—give your liver a break.

When you drink alcohol, your body relies on it for energy, instead of burning fat.

It will also make you search for food to nibble on.

What is a glass of wine?

It's pasta in a glass!!

(Do you *really* want that chardonnay now?)

SUPPORTING YOUR LIVER

This is a reflexology technique that can help support your liver.

- Hold your right hand with your left hand.

- With a gentle circular motion use the thumb of your left hand to massage the palm of your right hand.

- Do this for 2 minutes.

- Repeat twice daily.

GET THAT LIVER ENERGY MOVING

Place your finger on the skin between your big toe and the second toe. Pressing gently, move your finger up toward your ankle. You will feel a small dip about two inches up. Gently press this point for a minute to help promote the liver.

This is a strong acupressure point, Liv-3, that when activated helps rebalance the liver.

Whenever possible, eat foods
in their natural state

An apple . . .

not apple pie!

This will put less stress on your
liver and give you more energy.

As you eat healthier and
exercise more frequently, your
body will clear out toxins.

You will find that you have more energy.

You will look younger and more vibrant.

You will feel better—
emotionally and physically.

QUICK TOXIN RELEASE EXERCISE

There is a spot in the dip below your collarbone and next to your shoulder, which can feel slightly sensitive when touched. This is known as the sore spot.

Sore Spot

Rubbing this spot in a circular motion on each side of your body will activate an acupressure meridian that helps to release lymphatic congestion and clear out waste from your body.

Fewer toxins = more energy

Using the Power
of Your Mind

Self-hypnosis

If this section makes you nervous, relax!

This is not something you have to learn.

You are actually already an expert at self-hypnosis.

Your mind uses automatic trances—which is another term for self-hypnosis—to lock you into repeating certain behaviors.

When you're in this state, your conscious mind gets a break.

More often than not, these trances are among the many ways that our brains look after us—enabling us to function while simultaneously giving us a rest. Your thoughts can wander while you drive for miles on the same highway, and you automatically brush your teeth every morning, sometimes when you're only barely awake.

But automatic trances can also cause problems. They can keep you stuck in negative patterns, without you even realizing it's happening.

Your automatic food trances

Have you ever found yourself looking at an empty packet of food that you ate without tasting, without even noticing?

You were in a trance.

You mind has trances that it will lock you into, causing you to repeat behavior.

Shopping in the supermarket and automatically picking up the same brands of toilet paper or peanut butter, zoning out while watching TV . . .

. . . or eating the contents of the fridge when you're stressed.

After eating the food you find yourself "waking up" and becoming aware of what you have done. This can happen to smokers, and it is just as much of a problem for binge eaters.

Break your trance

In order to regain control you need to break this trance. Do something that your mind doesn't expect.

Wake your mind up!

Before your deeper mind takes over there is a moment when you can break out of your trance—a moment just before you stuff your face with food you don't need.

To do this, try:

Star jumps   **Stomping your feet**

Clapping your hands   **Shouting at yourself**

The first time you break the trance it will feel difficult, but each subsequent time you do, you are weakening the power it has over you.

Positive trances

It is possible to use the power of a trance to help you achieve your weight-loss goal.

You can harness the power of your mind and get it to work for you. This is a positive trance, and an empowering form of self-hypnosis.

How does this work?

When your mind imagines something over and over again it begins to believe that it has really happened.

We have all had the experience of waking up from a dream and not knowing whether it was real or not. Similarly, if your mind has repeatedly imagined that you are slim and healthy, it will look for ways of making this a reality.

By using mindfulness you have already practiced putting yourself into a wonderfully calming trancelike state. This is the beginning of self-hypnosis.

IMAGINING YOUR GOAL

Visualizing your goal vividly in your mind is extremely powerful. This vision will function like a huge magnet in your future, pulling you toward it—giving you the confidence and determination to achieve your target weight.

Read through the rest of the page and then allow your imagination to create a powerful vision of how it will feel to achieve a slimmer, healthier body. Use the technique of mindfulness (see pages 45–48) to help you relax.

Allow your mind to quiet down as you begin to focus on your breathing.

While in this relaxed state simply allow yourself to imagine that you have achieved your goal.

You are wearing the clothes you want to wear. Notice how people are responding to this new, slimmer you—how wonderful it feels to go about your day in this slim, healthy body.

Imagine shopping for clothes and choosing to try something on in exactly the right size for this slimmer you. Feel the sensation of the clothes as you put them on—feel how they skim over your body and fit you wonderfully.

Perhaps you catch sight of yourself in the mirror, and notice just how good you look.

Enjoy this feeling. Now notice the date on the calendar—this is the date you are going to achieve your goal by.

You find yourself smiling because you know that this is going to happen.

Now open your eyes.

REHEARSAL OF AN EVENING OUT

When you are at home you can be in control of what you are eating. But when you go out for dinner, it might feel as if you have been thrown into deep water and don't know how to swim. You may feel waves of anxiety hitting you as you see the amount and variety of food that is on offer before you.

First, use the technique of mindfulness to quiet your thoughts.

Once you feel calm and inwardly focused, allow yourself to imagine that you are getting ready to go out. You can visualize the evening unfolding as clearly as if you were watching it on film.

* Imagine arriving at the restaurant where you will be eating. See yourself sitting down at the table. You are composed and confident.

- Notice how you choose food and drinks that will help you achieve your goal of a slimmer you.

- You feel in control. It seems so easy to choose healthy food.

- Notice how you stop eating when you are no longer hungry—putting your knife and fork down and perhaps allowing food to be left on your plate.

- At the end of the meal you feel happy, relaxed, and satisfied.

- Open your eyes.

Repeat this exercise several times before going out for a meal.

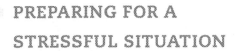

PREPARING FOR A
STRESSFUL SITUATION

Sometimes you know that an upcoming event is going to cause you stress. It might be the situation itself—perhaps a formal work outing, or a presentation—or perhaps it's the people who will surround you and the prospect of having to spend time with someone you don't really get along with.

Even if you can't control the event that causes the stress, by using self-hypnosis you *can* reduce the effect that it is going to have on you and your eating pattern. You can teach that deeper part of your mind how you want to behave.

- Come to a calm and inwardly focused state using mindfulness, and allow yourself to picture the situation.

- Watch yourself as you go through the entire event—from your preparation for it until you come home.

- As you do this, allow the tranquillity that you are experiencing in this state of mindfulness to change how you imagine yourself feeling and behaving during the event.

- Observe how this sense of calm allows you to respond differently to people.

- Run through the event in your mind several times, allowing for a variety of potentially stressful scenarios. Picture yourself responding with control, ease, and grace.

- Notice how calmly you are able to cope.

- Open your eyes.

Each time you carry this exercise out you might find that you respond in even better, calmer ways to the situation. And when it comes to the actual event, you will find yourself feeling collected, relaxed, and able to cope well.

The Wonders of Exercise

Many of my overweight clients have a gym membership and come into their first session saying that they hate the gym but they are going to start going regularly after seeing me.

I ask, "Why?"

If you hate the gym, please quit paying the fees!

There are so many other types of exercise you could be doing.

Walking	**Cycling**
Swimming	**Yoga**
Running	**Tennis**
Dancing	**Sailing**
Rowing	**Judo**
Pilates	**Aerobics**

You just need to find the activity that you enjoy. Otherwise you are not going to keep doing it.

Exercise:

Burns calories—when you exercise you are burning **extra** calories, which will help you reach your weight goals.

Boosts metabolism—this means you will continue burning calories even when you have finished exercising.

Makes your brain happy—as you exercise you release endorphins, which make you feel good.

Gets you into shape—exercise can help prevent heart disease and strokes, lower blood pressure, improve bone density, and reduce the risk of diabetes.

Does this sound familiar?

My metabolism is slowing down.

I'm getting older.

I can't lose weight.

Rubbish!

In reality you are probably doing less load-bearing exercise, and as a result, you have much less muscle mass—*this* is what is causing your metabolism to slow down.

The best way to speed it back up?

Get moving!

Your metabolism

. . . is not fixed.
. . . can change with what you eat and with exercise.

Keep dieting and you will keep gaining weight.

When your diet is restrictive and you skip meals, your body thinks that it is in a time of famine—and this makes your metabolism slow down in order to conserve energy.

Stop starving your body.

Eat to lose weight!

Water Water Water

If you are dehydrated:

Your metabolism will slow down.

Your body will feel tired.

You will have a false sensation of hunger.

Before you reach for that snack,
drink a glass of water!

Exercising can double
your metabolic rate.

But you must be exercising
enough to get sweaty
and out of breath!

GET THAT STUCK ENERGY MOVING!

Your brain is a center of energy, and sometimes it needs a boost.

If you are feeling sluggish, it's probably because you need to get this energy moving.

Your head is covered in acupressure points that, when massaged, will invigorate your mind and body.

- Sit somewhere comfortable.

- Become aware of your breathing as you inhale and exhale deeply and slowly. Imagine that you can follow the path of your breath as you do this.

- Begin massaging your forehead, cheeks and— gently—around the eyes. (A)

- Now, gently begin to massage your scalp with your fingertips, slowly continuing down to the base of your neck. (B, C, D)

- Finally, run your fingers down your neck to your shoulders and relax your hands. (E, F)

- While breathing deeply, take a few moments to notice any changes in how you are now feeling.

BOOSTING YOUR IMMUNE SYSTEM

When you are feeling stronger in mind and body you will have more energy for exercise.

This acupressure exercise can help to reinforce your immune system:

- Place your fingers on the points that stick out on your collarbone.

- Just below these, on the top part of your chest, you will feel slight depressions.

- Firmly press these points as you breathe deeply for one minute.

In acupressure, this is known as the K-27 point.

When you do something for 6 weeks it becomes a habit

Do something for 3 months and it will become a way of life.

What does this mean for you?

At first it might be difficult to put in place that new way of eating or new exercise regime.

But persist—in just a few short weeks you will find it becomes easier, and very soon it will become effortless—simply a part of your daily routine.

You will find yourself *automatically* eating better and exercising more.

TAPPING INTO YOUR METABOLISM

Helping you spark your metabolism

Follow the points on the tapping map and do one full circuit for each affirmation. Repeat each statement out loud as you tap.

For further reference, please see the tapping map on page 9.

- Even though I feel my metabolism has been slow, I am okay.

- I can let go of whatever has been slowing down my metabolism.

- I can allow my metabolism to speed up.

- I can feel energy beginning to pump through my body; my body is burning more calories.

- My metabolism is now speeding up to the perfect rate for me.

Note: This exercise should be done in the morning; if carried out at night it may affect sleep.

Step to it

Sedentary people walk less than 5,000 steps a day.

Active people walk about 10,000 steps a day.

Get a pedometer!!!

It has been shown that wearing a pedometer will help
increase the number of steps you take each day.

**Just a few extra steps a day
could make a huge difference to
your life and your health.** *

*As discussed in "How many steps a day are enough? Preliminary
pedometer indices for public health," by C. Tudor-Locke and
D.R. Bassett, Jr., *Sports Medicine,* Vol. 34, No. 1, 1–8, 2004.

Exercise releases
tension and stress.

Exercise also releases
endorphins—those wonderful
mood-boosting chemicals.

So after a workout, you feel
calmer and happier!

When you are happier, you
eat healthier and eat less.

TAPPING OUT NEGATIVE EXERCISE THOUGHTS

Helping you feel energized and motivated

Follow the points on the tapping map and do one full circuit for each affirmation. Repeat each statement out loud as you tap.

For further reference, please see the tapping map on page 9.

- Even though I don't really feel like exercising, I am okay.

- Even though I don't want to go and exercise, I am okay.

- I am tired and I accept myself.

- Even though I am worried I haven't got the energy to exercise, I am okay.

- Even though I find exercising difficult, I accept myself.

- Even though it is scary to change, I am okay.

To conclude this exercise, repeat the last statement while gently rubbing the sore spot.

Finally finish by tapping the Karate Chop point 8 times.

STILL FEELING NEGATIVE
ABOUT EXERCISE?

Tapping will help you shift those negative emotions.

Begin tapping at your temple, following the skin behind the ears and down the sides of your neck, ending as you reach the tops of your shoulders.*

Left-hand side:

As you tap, repeat this phrase 5 times:

I am no longer negative when I think about exercise.

Right-hand side:

As you tap, repeat this phrase 5 times:

I enjoy exercise. When I exercise I feel great.

*Developed by George Goodheart, the founder of applied kinesiology, and Donna Eden, author of *Energy Medicine for Women*.

WANT TO EXERCISE—BUT FEELING SLUGGISH?

This energy tap will give you a mental and physical boost, helping you to find the energy and motivation to exercise:

- Start by breathing deeply in and out through your nose.
- Place your fingers on your forehead and gently massage the skin. (A)
- Continue to gently massage your temples. (B)
- Now use all 10 fingers to tap across the top of your scalp, like raindrops. (C)
- Using your index fingers, tap on the inside edge of your eyebrows 8 times. (D)
- Repeat on the outside edge of your eyes and then under each eye. (E)
- Now tap on the top of your lip and then on your chin, again tapping about 8 times in each location. (F)
- Lastly, gently rub your sore spot for about 30 seconds.
- Shake out your hands and arms to finish.

Remember that you will have slip-ups—you are not perfect

You are only human.

When you accept this you don't have to waste energy beating yourself up about mistakes. You don't have to give up on your plan for the day or week just because you were running late and had a muffin for breakfast— you can shrug it off and nudge yourself back onto your correct path.

Spending less energy worrying means you have more energy for the activities that make you healthier!

Boost your oxygen levels to boost your weight loss

- Each time you exhale you breathe out toxins.
- By breathing deeply you are stimulating your lymphatic system, which helps to remove even more toxins from your body.
- Deep breathing provides the cells of your body with oxygen, especially your intestines, and it promotes your body's ability to absorb nutrients.

Breathing seems like the most natural, effortless thing we do. But paying attention to how we breathe is very important. Breathing deeply can boost your metabolism, while also giving you more energy for exercise. As a result, you will burn more calories.

- Breathing deeply can boost your metabolism.
- This means you will burn more calories!

Most of us, however, take only shallow breaths. When you are shallow breathing, only the top of your chest will move. But when you are breathing deeply, the top of your chest will be still, and your stomach will move in and out.

To access your deep breathing, imagine that as you inhale, you are following the air as it travels down into your stomach and following the same breath out again as you exhale. Try to take 10 deep breaths like this 3 times a day for maximum benefit.

BREATHING DEEPER

Simply focusing on your breathing can give you an instant boost.

- Stand up.

- Make one hand into a fist and place it gently at the bottom of your ribs.

- Place your other hand on top of the fist and gently pull in.

- Inhale deeply through your nose, feeling the pressure of your breath against your hands. Relax your fist as you exhale through your mouth.

- Repeat 10 times.

You will feel a surge of energy in mind and body.

SECTION 9

Achieving Your Goal

Your goal is to lose weight—to become that slim, healthy you that you have dreamt about for so long.

In order to achieve your goal it is important to stay focused on what you want, and to know where you are going.

It is also important to understand the blocks to weight loss that might be standing in your way. If you can begin to recognize these obstacles, then you can consciously face them and overcome them.

How will you know when you have reached your goal?

Is it by the number on the scale?
How many miles you are able to run?
Fitting into a certain pair of jeans?

When do you want to achieve your goal?

In a month? 6 months? 12 months?

Take some time to think about
this and set a realistic date.

If you don't know where you are going
you are never going to get there.

What is stopping you?

What has been preventing you from losing that excess weight?

Imagine you have reached your goal: you are the size, weight, and shape that you want to be.

Just close your eyes and experience this for a few minutes. Imagine being in that body. Take the time to be fully aware of what it is like to be in this new body.

How does it *really* feel to be this size?

* Do you have any negative emotions about being this size?
* Is there anything you have promised yourself you will do when you are this slim?
* Anything you might be nervous about actually doing?
* Is there anyone in your life who is not happy about what you have achieved or about the way you look?

Think about how you would deal with any negativity that arises once you have achieved your goal. If you are prepared for a negative reaction then it will not set you back. You will be able to deflect it and feel happy within yourself.

Promises

Take a few moments to think about the things you have promised yourself you will do when you are slim.

You might have vowed that you'll buy new clothes or finally try a new haircut.

Or you might have promised yourself that you will make a bigger change:

- Go back to school and enroll in the course you have always wanted to take.
- Get a new job—one that really challenges you or that you are more passionate about.
- Start dating again.

Sometimes we promise ourselves things that we really truly want, but that also make us a bit nervous.

If you are aware that there is something you might be nervous about doing once you are slim, then you can take action now toward becoming more confident about whatever it is that you want to do. Take small steps to achieve your big goal—get a brochure for that college course, talk to a recruiter about possible career moves, or ask a friend to start thinking about which of their single acquaintances they could set you up with.

Are you comfortable with change?

As you lose weight and move toward that new body shape, the shape you have always wanted, you are creating change.

These changes in yourself—how you feel and how you look—may also lead to changes in how you are perceived and treated by others.

Change can cause you to feel nervous, and you may want to retreat back into the familiar.

This means gaining back the weight you have lost.

This may make you feel safe again—and it may have happened in the past without your even realizing what was going on.

But now that you are becoming more aware of how your mind and body are connected, you are learning new ways of being, enabling you to cope with the anxieties that change awakens. You can embrace the new slimmer, healthier, happier you with confidence.

If you are not comfortable with the new you, no one else will be.

Becoming comfortable with the new you is very important.

You deserve to enjoy this new slimmer you.

Negative people

It's hard to imagine that there would be people in your life who might respond negatively to your weight loss.

But there might be.

Being aware of what is causing that negative emotion will help you to overcome it—and to feel confident about what you are achieving for yourself.

- Sometimes friends can feel threatened by the "new you" and will want to push you back into that old shape so they'll feel comfortable in their life again.
- Partners can be jealous of the attention your new slimmer figure might attract. Or they may worry that you might leave them as your confidence grows.
- Family members—mothers, fathers, siblings—may also make negative comments about your new look. Your weight loss might be highlighting their own insecurities.

TAPPING OUT BLOCKS TO WEIGHT LOSS

Helping you move forward to a slimmer you

Follow the points on the tapping map and do one full circuit for each affirmation. Repeat each statement out loud as you tap.

For further reference, please see the tapping map on page 9.

- Even though I am nervous about being slim, I am okay.

- There may be reasons why I haven't let myself be slim before, but I can choose to let those go now.

- I can allow myself to move on.

- I am stronger now, and I can enjoy being slimmer.

- I am not the person I was—I am more confident now, and I accept myself.

- I can allow myself to be slim and happy.

- I can allow myself to reach my goal.

Set the date you will achieve your goal

Put the date you are going to achieve your goal onto your calendar.

Think about the changes that are already starting to happen in your life that will allow you to easily achieve this goal.

You might need to put in some other dates of smaller milestones you want to reach that will keep you moving toward this ultimate objective.

As you approach this date, keep checking on your progress. Continue making the changes you need to in order to achieve the results you want, when you want them.

Smile—you can feel good about yourself.

You are changing, you are making this happen.

You are important.

You are important.

You are important.

Get it?

What if you are important?

Then it is important that you look after yourself.

It is important that you pay attention to how you are feeling.

If you are important, then you give yourself time to exercise.

If you are important, then every morsel that goes into your body matters.

This is not a diet—
this is a change of lifestyle

You may slip off your path occasionally, but when you do, remember it's okay—pick up *The Little Book of Diet Help,* and there will be assistance and encouragement waiting.

You deserve to be happy and slim,
and you can be.

Acknowledgments

I would like to thank my agent, Darley Anderson, and his team, especially Sophie Gordon, who believed in this book, and Clare Wallace, who is amazing.

I would also like to thank Sarah Cantin, who is a tireless and wonderful editor.

Thanks also must go to all my family, my husband, Michael, and my daughters, Rosie and Molly, for their love and understanding.

About the Author

I am a therapist based in England with practices in Sheffield and London. I use a combination of therapies (hypnotherapy, EFT, and NLP) to help adults, teens, and children with a wide range of issues.

I also run Hyp-Slim weight-loss courses. These workshops incorporate hypnosis, along with all the techniques used in this book, to help people lose weight naturally and permanently.

A number of years ago BC (Before Children), I completed a PhD in chemistry and conducted research at various universities.

After having children I decided that a career change was in order. What I really wanted was to see a life coach, but at the time I couldn't afford one. So I did the next best thing, and trained to become one myself! This led me into a world of therapy and self-help that, as a skeptical scientist, I had avoided for years. But this world has completely changed my life—for the better. I hope that with *The Little Book of Diet Help* as your guide, it will change yours too.

Kimberly Willis
www.kimberlywillis.co.uk

Printed in the United States
By Bookmasters